Dr. Ben's
Dental Guide

A Visual Reference to Teeth, Dental Conditions and Treatment

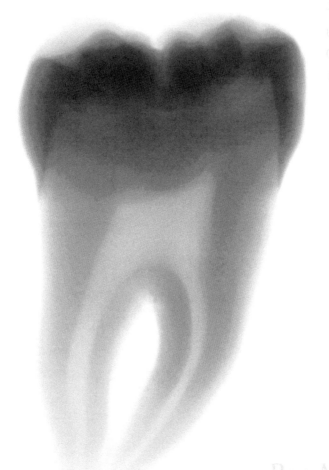

Ben Magleby, D.D.S.

This is a visual reference book explaining many of the different aspects and restorative options for teeth.

No brand names for products and services were used in this book.

Illustrations were hand drawn and colored digitally.

For coloring pages, worksheets and additional information on dental health, visit

www.sugarbugdoug.com

ISBN-13: 978-1494841256
ISBN-10: 1494841258

Printed by KDP, an Amazon.com company

This book is a
collection of diagrams,
x-rays and pictures
to explain common
dental conditions
and treatment.

I hope that you
will find this
helpful in making
choices about
your dental health.

Ben Magleby, D.D.S.

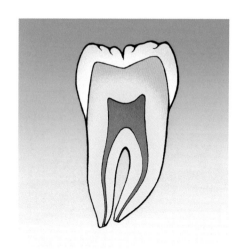

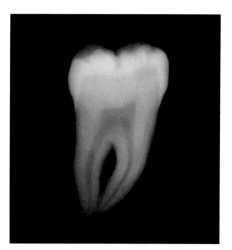

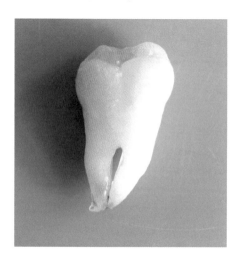

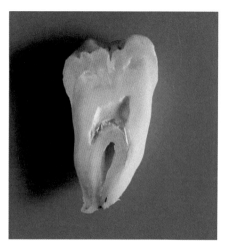

As you read
through this
book, look for
pictures that
correlate.

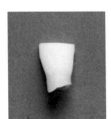

For Ian, Max and Zack
...who make me smile every day.

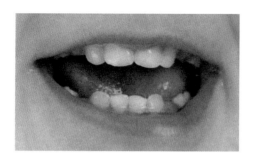

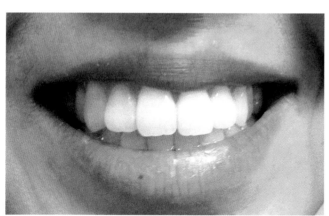

Table of Contents

Teeth

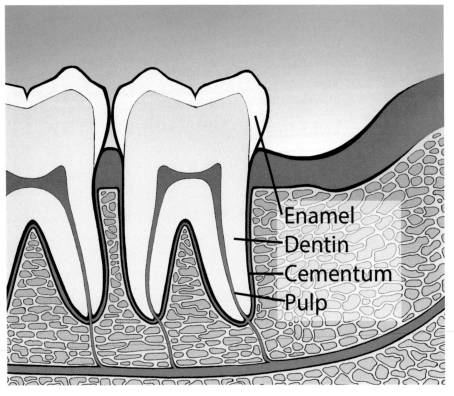

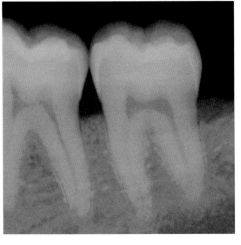

Enamel
Dentin
Cementum
Pulp

Teeth are made of 4 main materials: enamel, dentin, cementum and pulp. **Enamel** makes up the outside of the crown and is the strongest material made by your body. **Dentin** makes up most of the inside of the tooth and the root. The root is covered with **cementum**, a thin coating that makes the attachment to bone stronger. The **pulp** is made up of nerves and blood vessels.

There are four different types of teeth

Incisors - used for cutting food and speaking

Canines/Cuspids - used for tearing food and protecting the teeth around them

Bicuspids/ Premolars - help to chew food

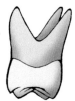

Molars - used for grinding food

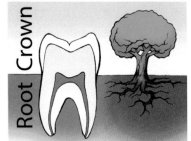

Root | Crown

Just like trees have roots under the ground, teeth have roots under the gums. They support the tooth and hold it in place. The part above the gums is called the crown.

Primary/Deciduous/Baby Teeth - 20

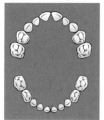

A child's first primary incisors will grow in when they are about 6 months old. Their last set of primary molars will grow in when they are about 2 years old.

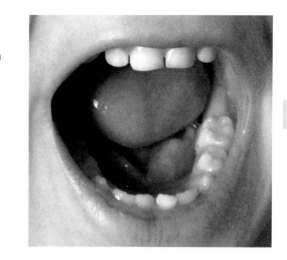

Mixed Dentition

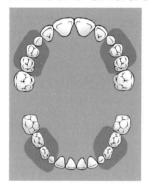

By the time a child is 8 years old, they will usually have replaced the 8 incisors in the front of their mouth. When a child is about 12 years old, they will usually have replaced most of the other 12 primary teeth.

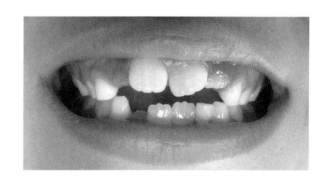

Permanent/Adult Teeth - 32

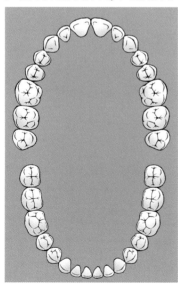

The first permanent teeth erupt when a child is about 6 years old. These are usually the first molars. They often come in just before the lower central incisors are replaced. The last set of permanent teeth are also molars. The wisdom teeth erupt at about 17-21 years of age.

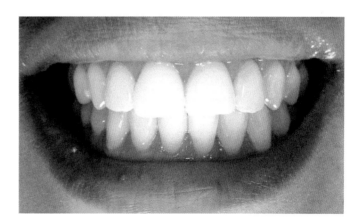

Dental Hygiene

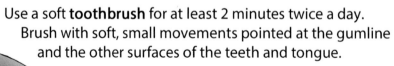

Use a soft **toothbrush** for at least 2 minutes twice a day. Brush with soft, small movements pointed at the gumline and the other surfaces of the teeth and tongue.

Electric toothbrushes usually come with built-in timers and brush with soft, small movements automatically. This makes it much easier to keep teeth clean.

Proxy brushes or **interdental brushes** are used for cleaning under bridges, braces and between teeth that may have larger spacing.

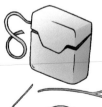

Floss is used to clean between teeth. There are also threaders that can be used to get the floss into difficult areas, like under bridges or around braces. Another type of floss comes in pre-cut sections with a built-in threader and a thicker section for better cleaning.

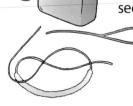

Floss holders come in many different styles, some are disposable while others are meant to be reused.

A **dental water jet** or **water flosser** sprays a stream of water or mouthwash that can be used to clean between teeth and around dental appliances.

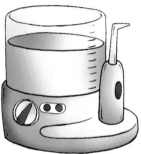

A **tongue scraper** helps to remove plaque from the tongue.

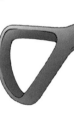

When evaluating **toothpaste** and **mouthwash**, choose a product based on active ingredients and personal needs. In toothpaste, notice the amount of fluoride, antibiotics and anti-hypersensitivity medication. In mouthwash, notice how much alcohol, fluoride and other ingredients.

When applying toothpaste, a little is enough. This is especially true of children who may accidently swallow it.

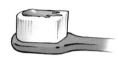

Drinking **water** after eating and throughout the day is a good way to help a mouth stay healthy.

Sugarless gum helps to clean teeth. Some sugarless gum is sweetened with xylitol, a sugar that stops the growth of cavity forming bacteria.

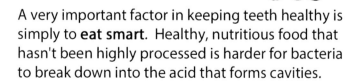

A very important factor in keeping teeth healthy is simply to **eat smart**. Healthy, nutritious food that hasn't been highly processed is harder for bacteria to break down into the acid that forms cavities.

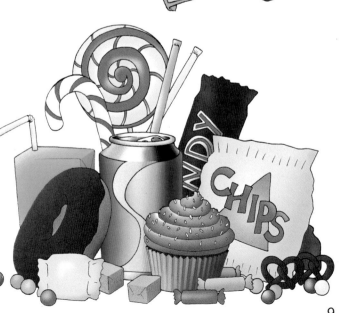

Frequent snacking on food full of simple carbohydrates feeds these bacteria much too often. This is one of the fastest ways to grow tooth decay.

Gum Disease

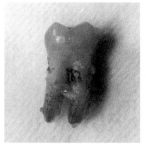

Healthy Gingiva

Gingivitis

Periodontitis

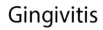

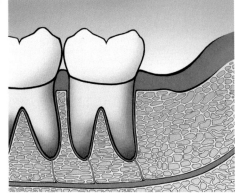
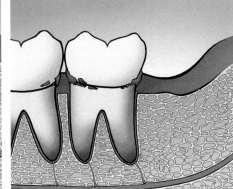
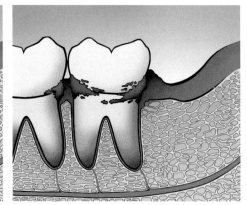

Gum disease starts out as plaque buildup around the gumline and causes the gums to become infected and inflamed. This infection is called **gingivitis** and later, **periodontitis**. While gum disease does not damage the tooth itself, this infection causes the supporting gums and bone to be destroyed. If plaque stays for a long time, it turns into **calculus** (also known as tartar) and can grow deeper and deeper down the side of the root. As it grows deeper, the more painful the gums are and the looser teeth become until they fall out.

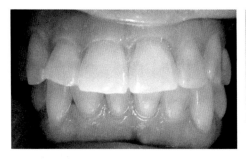
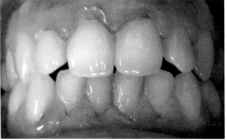
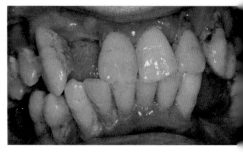

One way to see how healthy gums are is to notice the color. When gums are pink, that usually means they are very healthy. The more infected they are, the more inflamed, swollen and red they will become. They usually bleed a lot easier as well.

Calculus buildup below the gumline is much harder to clean and much more dangerous than calculus above the gumline. This buildup leads to bone loss, abscesses and tooth loss. It can also lead to more serious problems like systemic infection, heart disease and in pregnant women, low birth weight babies.

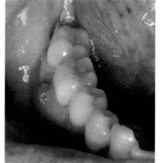
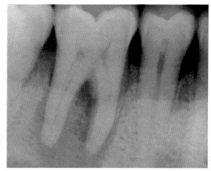

Advanced Periodontitis

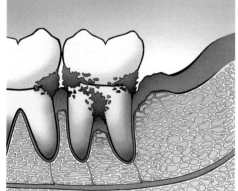
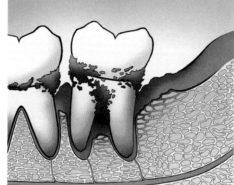
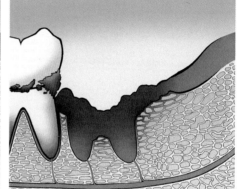

The small instrument that dentists use to measure gums is called a **perio probe**. Measurements help to find out where gum disease is and how to best treat it. Periodontal pocket measurements of 1-3 mm are good and 4-5 mm are worse. Measurements of 10 mm or more usually means that the tooth is unsaveable.

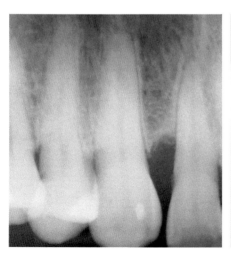
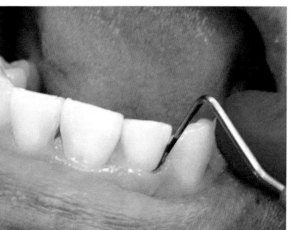
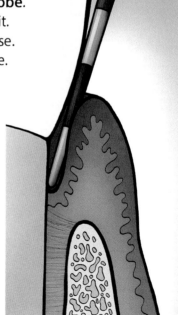

Cleaning

Prophy

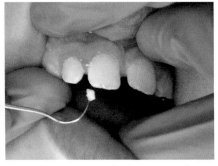 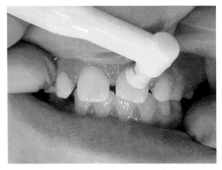

A prophylactic cleaning, or **prophy**, involves removing plaque and light calculus from above the gumline. It is usually done with a prophy cup, floss and hand scalers.

Scaling and Root Planing (SRP), Deep Cleaning

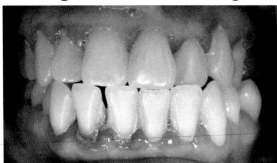 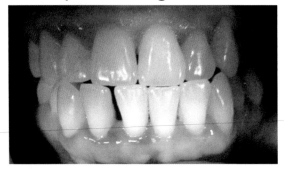

Scaling and root planing involves removing bacteria, plaque and calculus from below the gumline. This may require anesthesia. In addition to hand scalers, ultrasonic instruments can also be used to remove calculus and irrigate the gum tissue. Some of the calculus deposits can be very large.

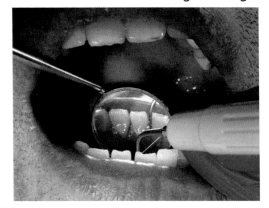 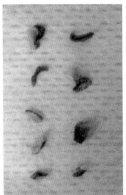 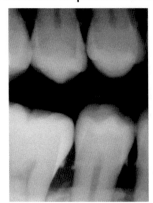 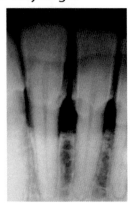

Gum Surgery

Periodontal Surgery

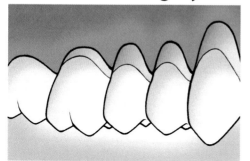

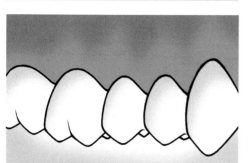

The main reason to have periodontal surgery is to make gum tissue easier to clean and maintain by reducing pocket depth.

Periodontal surgery can also:

- restore gum recession along sensitive areas
- fix a "gummy" smile
- play a part in placing and restoring implants
- correct impacted teeth
- remove suspicious lesions
- free up tissue that is too tight and restricting

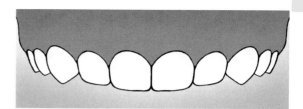

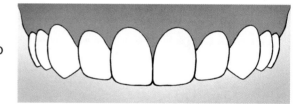

Crown Lengthening

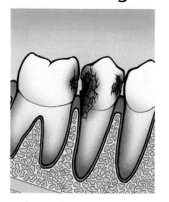
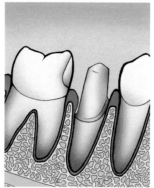
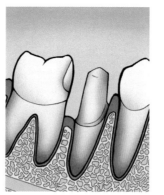
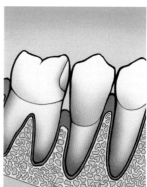

When the decay on a tooth extends near or below the level of the bone, then restoring the tooth requires crown lengthening. During the restoration process, the bone and gingiva are lowered so the tooth will not be permanently inflamed when the final restoration is placed.

Cavity

Tooth Decay, Rotten Teeth, Dental Caries

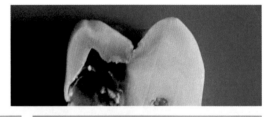

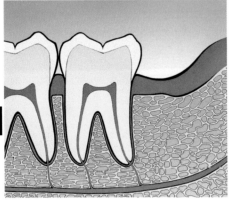 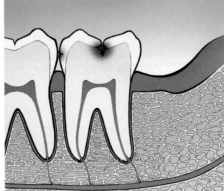 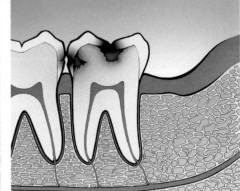

Whenever bacteria metabolize simple carbohydrates, they make acid as a waste product. When this acid stays on teeth, the teeth will slowly dissolve and rot. This leads to holes in the teeth, or cavities. As the cavities grow, teeth can become painful, break and fall out.

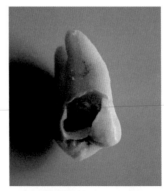

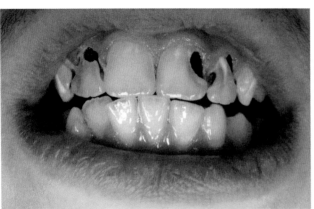 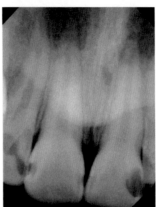 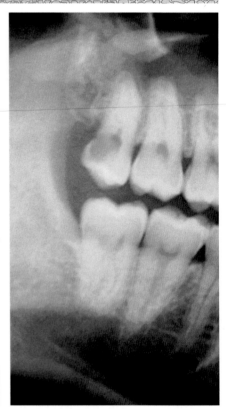

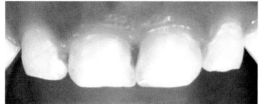
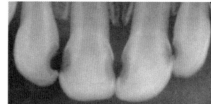

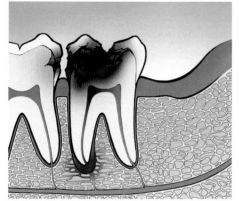
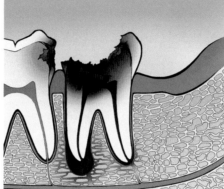
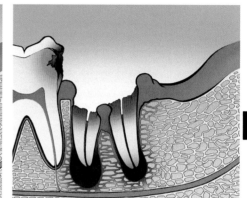

X-rays show cavities between teeth. They also show how deep the decay is.

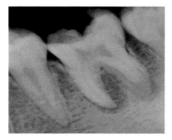

Cavities usually start out in areas that are hard to clean, like the central grooves, between teeth or around appliances.

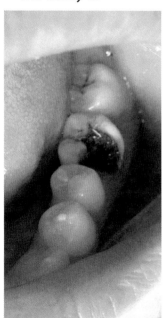

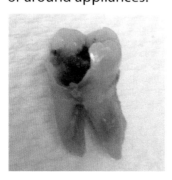

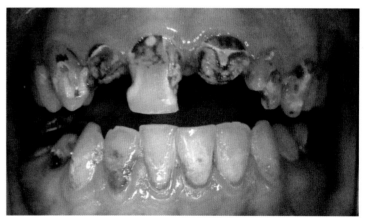

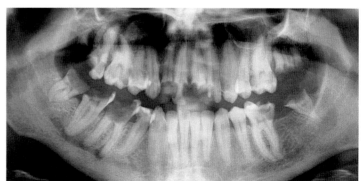

Filling
Amalgam, Composite, Sealant

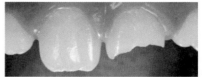 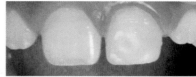

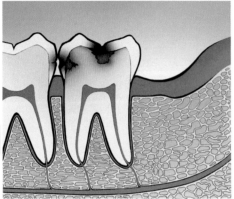 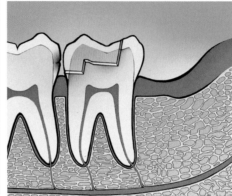 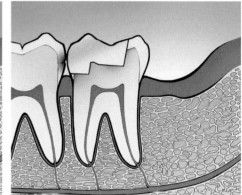

After removing the decay from a tooth, there needs to be something placed in the hole. There are several materials that can be used, including: silver amalgam, white composite, gold and porcelain. After any tooth is worked on, it is normal for that tooth to be sensitive for a little while. If the bite feels different when the anesthetic wears off, consult a dentist.

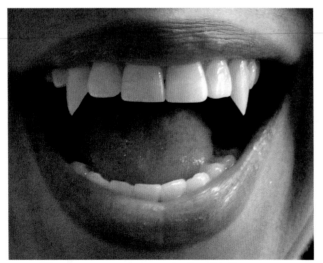

These were removed after Halloween.

Composite

Bonding these "white fillings" to teeth can solve many problems. Some applications include restoring broken teeth and cavities, bonding orthodontics and veneers, making sensitive areas less painful and a variety of cosmetic applications.

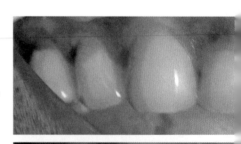

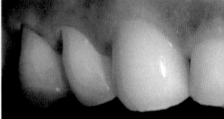

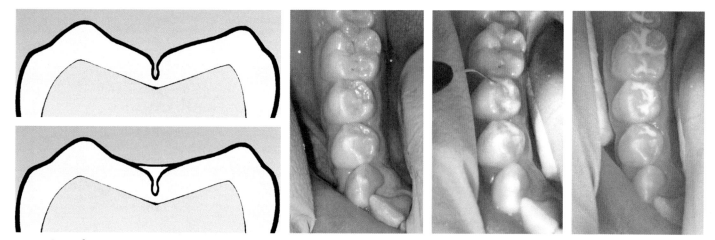

Sealant
Some teeth have deep grooves. These can be very difficult to clean and are one of the easiest places to grow decay. "Sealing" means to place a small filling in the grooves of a tooth.

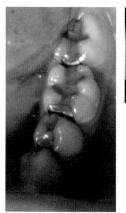
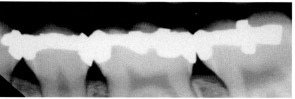

Amalgam
"Silver fillings" are another good option for restoring decay. Metal shows up bright white on x-rays.

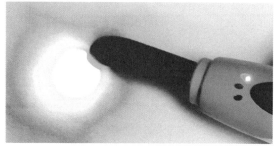

The blue light is used to "cure" or harden the composite material.

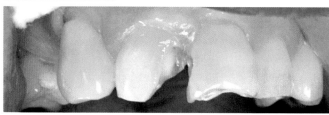
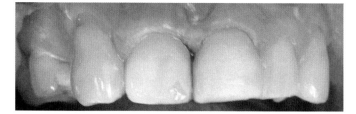
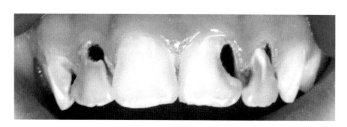
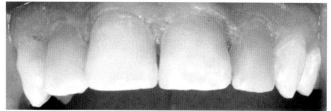

17

Root Canal
Endodontic Treatment

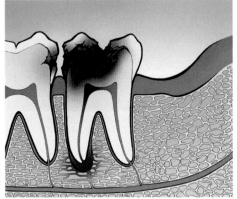 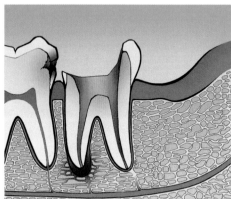 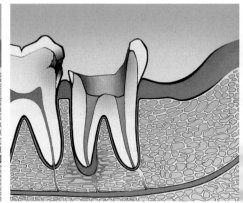

When the nerve of a tooth dies, then saving the tooth requires a root canal. Teeth usually die because of large cavities. They can also die from trauma. Root canals involve removing all of the decay and then removing the nerve of the tooth. Once the nerve chamber is cleaned and shaped, it is filled with a pink material called **guttapercha**.

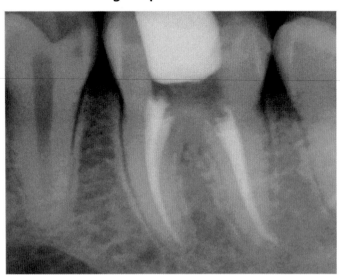

Even after a root canal is done, it may become infected and may need to be redone.

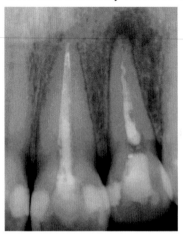 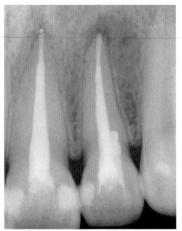

After a root canal is finished, many times a temporary filling is placed in the tooth. This needs to be replaced with a permanent filling.

Buildup

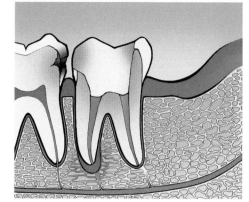

After the root canal is finished, the tooth needs a large filling called a **buildup** and a **crown**.

Post

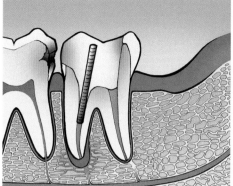

If there is not very much of the tooth remaining, then a **post** may be needed in one or more of the canals to help keep the buildup and crown in place.

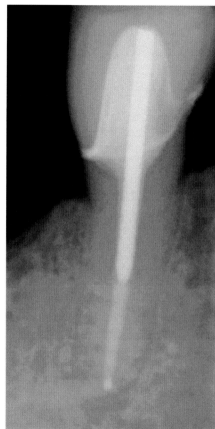

Crown

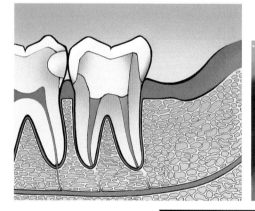

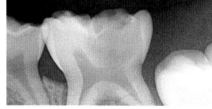

Primary teeth with big cavities can be saved just like permanent teeth.

Different materials are used, but the basic idea is still the same. Remove the infection and fill the space with something to keep bacteria and food out.

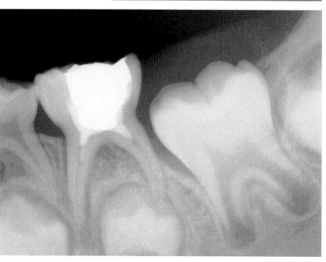

19

Crown
Cap, Bridge, Veneer, Inlay, Onlay, Partial Crown

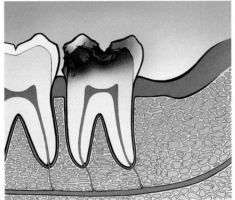 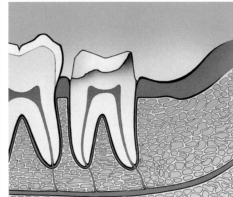 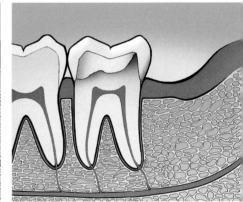

A crown is a type of dental restoration that covers the whole tooth. This is usually needed because of large decay or because the tooth is cracked. After the tooth is cleaned and shaped, an impression is taken so the crown can be made from a model of the tooth. This impression is made from a type of putty that sets around the tooth or from a specialized digital camera. After the crown is made, it is cemented or bonded to the tooth.

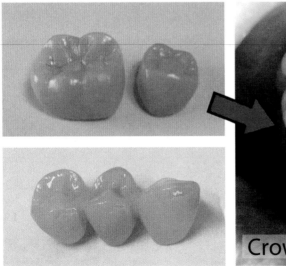 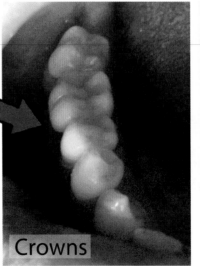

Crowns

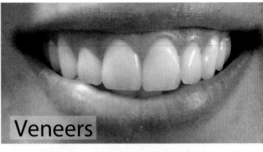

Veneers

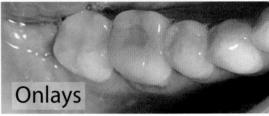

Onlays

Crown - Covers and protects the whole tooth.

Partial Crown/Inlay/Onlay - Restores part of the tooth. Uses the same material as a crown, so it is much stronger than a filling.

Veneer - Covers the front of the tooth, more for aesthetic reasons than to restore decay.

Bridge - Two or more crowns linked together, used to replace missing teeth.

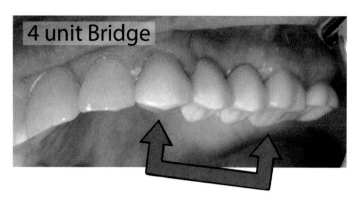

Materials

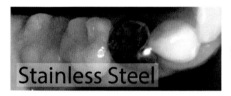

Stainless Steel - Usually used for primary teeth, inexpensive and not custom made.

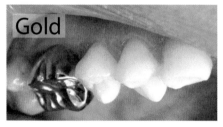

Gold - One of most durable materials used in dentistry.

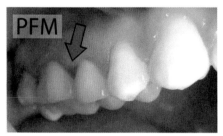

Porcelain Fused to Metal (PFM) - A metal core (usually gold) with porcelain baked on the outside. Sometimes the metal shows from under the porcelain. It can be also be fabricated to have a metal biting surface.

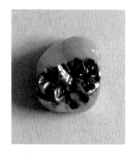

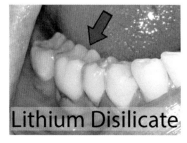

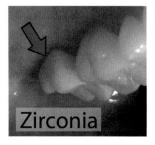

Full Ceramic - Tooth colored materials such as zirconia and lithium disilicate do not to need a metal backing. These can be used to fabricate the entire crown or have porcelain added to increase aesthetics. Some restorations can be fabricated in under an hour with digital impressions and CAD/CAM technology.

21

Implant

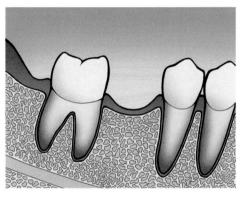 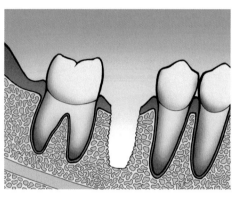 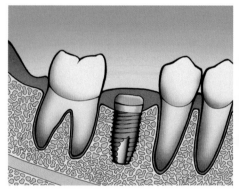

When a tooth is missing, one option is to replace it with an implant. After measurements are made, the implant is placed in the jaw and allowed to heal. Healing time varies greatly and can take up to 4-6 months. This time depends on how strong the bone is along with the implant's location in the mouth.

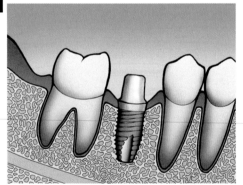 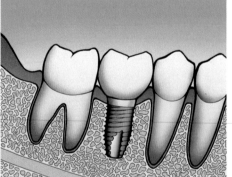

After the implant is secure in the bone, a small part is attached to the top of the implant called an **abutment**. An impression is taken of this abutment and a crown is made and attached.

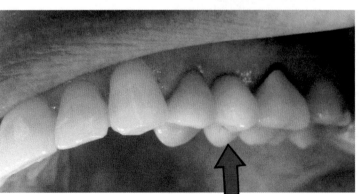 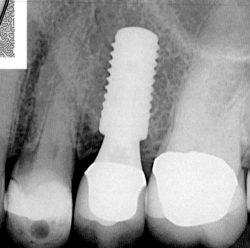

Implants are very versatile. In addition to replacing one tooth with an implant, several implants can be used together to support a bridge of many teeth. They can also be used to stabilize a denture or partial denture. Implants can even be used with braces to help move teeth.

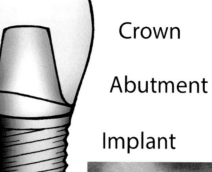

Crown

Abutment

Implant

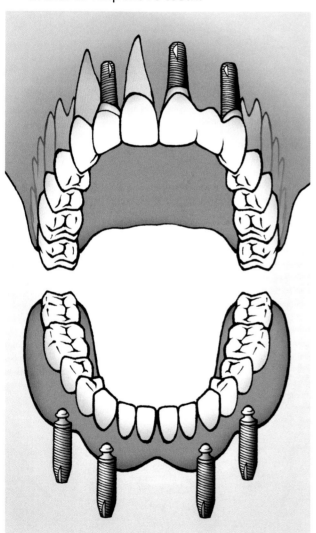

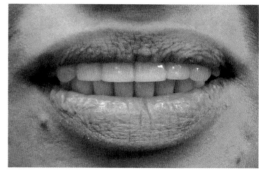

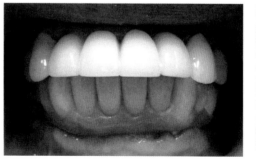

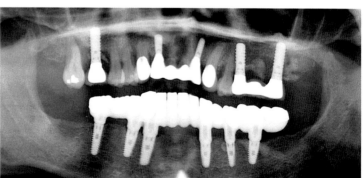

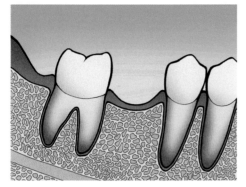

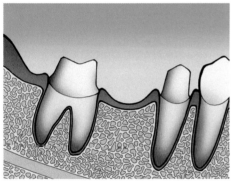

What is the difference between a bridge and an implant?

Bridge Attaches to Teeth

It usually takes 2 appointments that are about 2 weeks apart to finish a bridge. The first appointment is to prepare the teeth and take the impression, the second is to deliver the bridge.

Some tooth structure needs to be removed on the adjacent teeth to make room for the bridge. These teeth need to be structurally sound and be strong enough to handle the additional force.

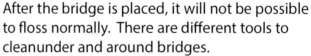

If either or both of these teeth have big cavities or fillings then placing a bridge will restore these teeth.

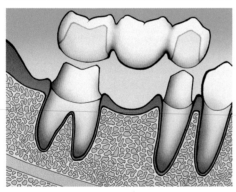

After the bridge is placed, it will not be possible to floss normally. There are different tools to cleanunder and around bridges.

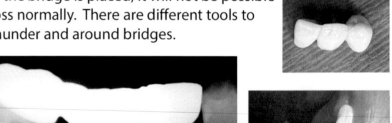

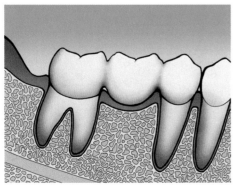

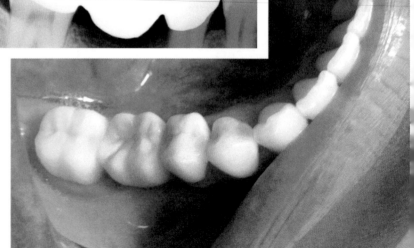

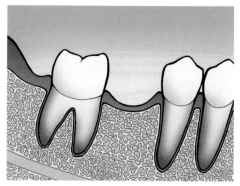

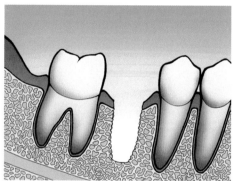

Implant Attaches to Bone

After placing an implant in the bone, there can be a healing time of up to 4-6 months before the crown can be placed.

No tooth structure needs to be removed to place an implant.

There needs to be good bone support for an implant. If there is not enough bone, additional surgery and healing time may be necessary. In some cases, a nerve or sinus may make this difficult.

Implants are usually more expensive than bridges.

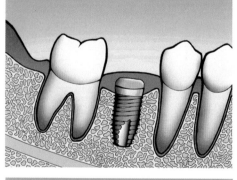

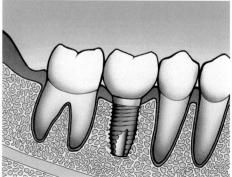

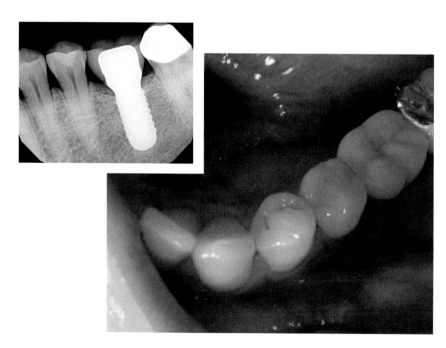

25

Denture
Removable Dental Appliances, False Teeth, Plates

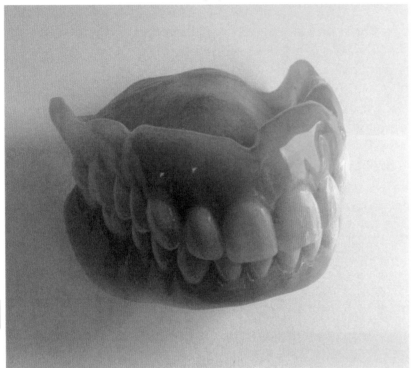
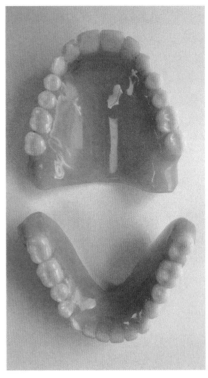

Full dentures and partial dentures are removable appliances that are worn to replace missing teeth. While full dentures stay in place with suction on the jaw, partial dentures can attach to remaining teeth to make them more secure.

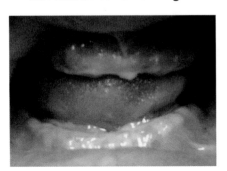
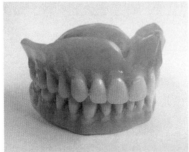
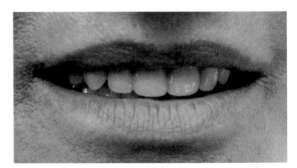

Both full and partial dentures can be supported with implants.

Partial Denture

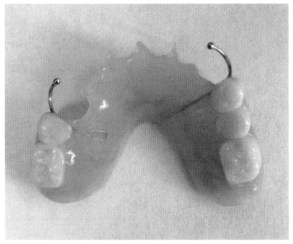

Stay Plate/Flipper - Fabricated out of acrylic and wire.

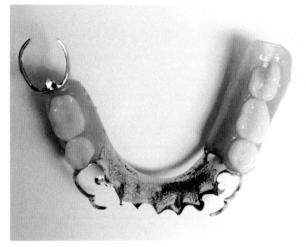

Cast Metal Framework - Acrylic on a custom cast metal frame.

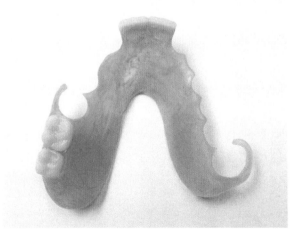

Flexible Partial - These are made from a thermoplastic nylon material.

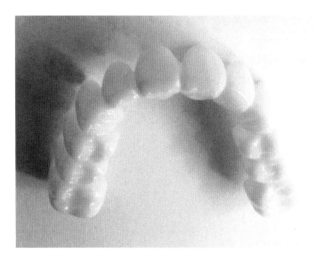

Full Arch Cosmetic Appliance - Covers the outside of all the teeth.

Removable partials can be a permanent solution or a temporary appliance.

Extraction
Removal of Teeth

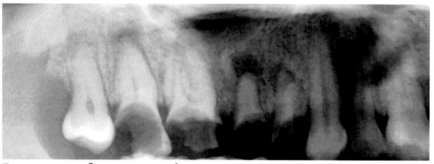
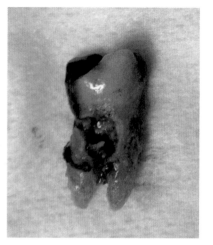

Reasons for a tooth extraction

The tooth cannot be saved or is very difficult to save.
- deep decay
- trauma
- periodontal disease

There may not be enough room.
- primary teeth in the way of permanent teeth
- extra teeth that are not needed
- permanent teeth are too crowded
- wisdom teeth that cannot be kept clean

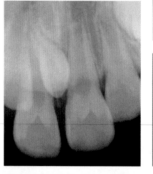
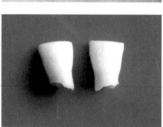

A treatment plan that involves dentures or orthodontics may call for extractions.

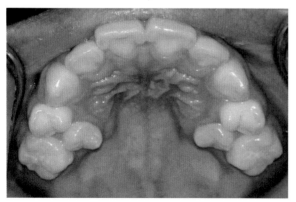
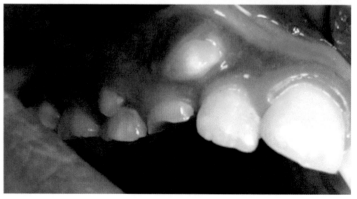

Options available after a tooth extraction

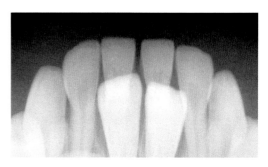

1. Leave the area open.

2. Move other teeth to fill in the space. Sometimes this happens naturally, sometimes orthodontics are needed to successfully position the teeth and close the space.

3. Denture - This can replace one or more teeth, this appliance is removable.

4. Bridge - This appliance is not removable, it is cemented to the teeth next to the open space.

5. Implant - This is also not removable, this attaches directly to the jaw.

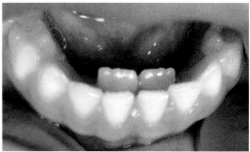

Bone Grafting - After a tooth extraction, the bone in the area will usually heal lower and thinner than it was when the tooth was present. This can create problems when restoring the area, especially when restoring with implants. Placing a bone graft in the extraction site will allow the area to heal without losing bone height and width.

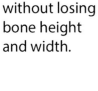

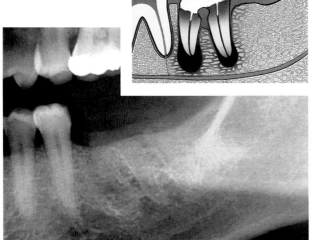

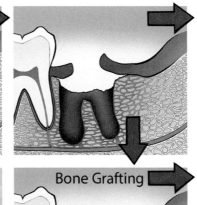

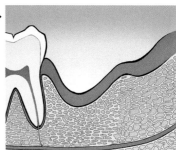

Bone Grafting

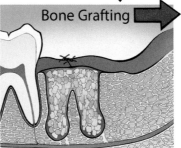

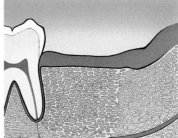

Wisdom Teeth
Third Molars

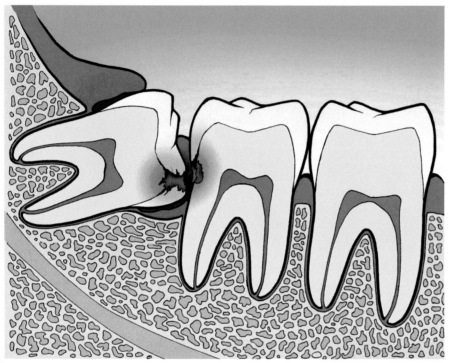

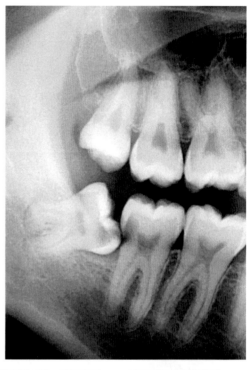

Wisdom teeth are a set of molars that people usually get when they are about 17-21 years old. They are like any other teeth, but sometimes they don't have enough room to come in all the way or can't come in straight. When this happens they are difficult to keep clean and can lead to gum disease and cavities.

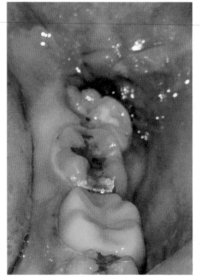

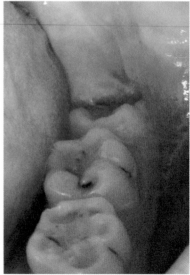

Some wisdom teeth are very simple to extract and will heal quickly with little or no swelling.

Other wisdom teeth need to be surgically removed. As a result, the healing process will take longer and most likely involve swelling.

Most extractions will heal within 2 weeks.

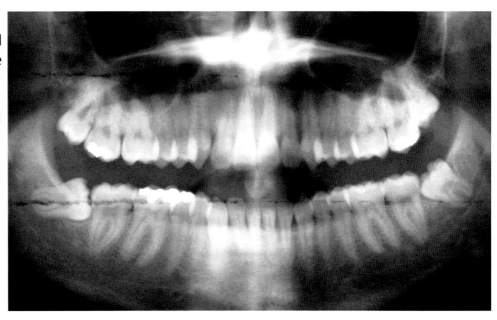

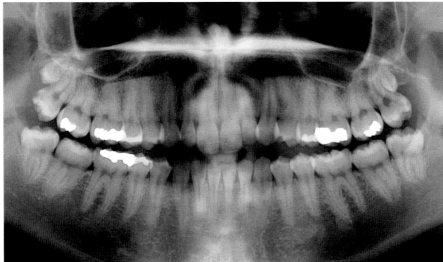

Most people have 4 wisdom teeth. While some may have 1, 2 or 3, others may have extra or none at all.

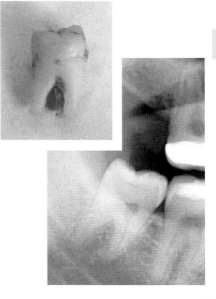

This person had 6.

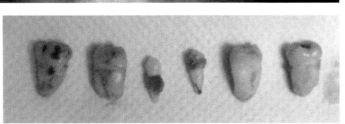

Braces
Orthodontics, Retainers, Space Maintainers

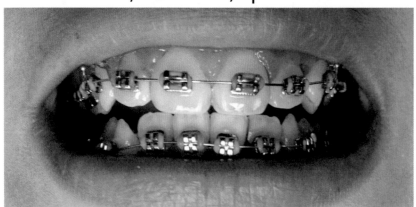 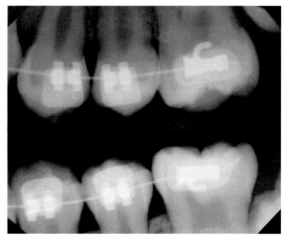

Braces can correct many types of problems: over and under bites, cross bites, spacing and crowding. Sometimes if teeth need to be extracted, braces can be used to move other teeth and fill in the space.

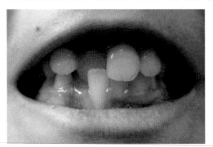 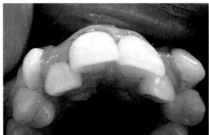 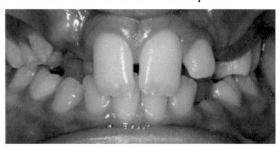

Teeth move whenever pressure is placed on them. As they grow in, teeth slowly drift according to the cheeks, tongue, other teeth and anything else that puts pressure on them. Braces and other orthodontic appliances can be used to move teeth or to keep them where they are.

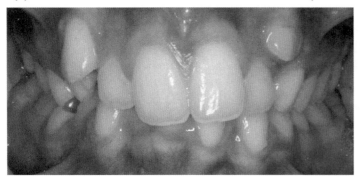 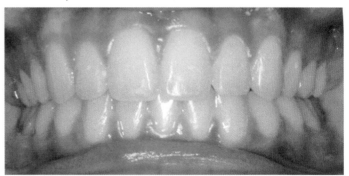

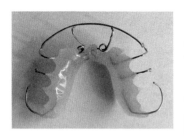

In addition to braces there are removable appliances that can also move teeth. Some are similar to retainers, others are clear aligners.

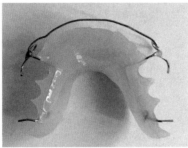

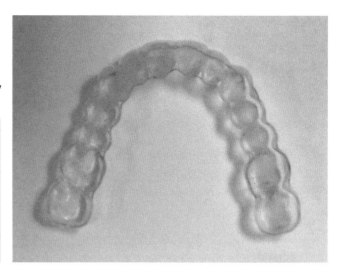

Retainers are appliances that hold teeth in the same position, usually at the end of treatment. They can be bonded to teeth or be removable.

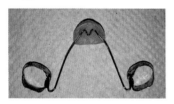

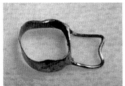

Space maintainers are cemented on teeth to keep them from moving. This retains the room for permanent teeth if a primary tooth is lost prematurely.

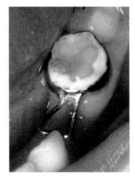

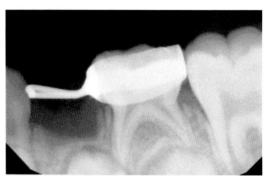

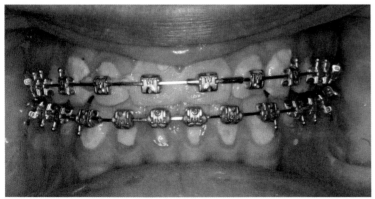

Good oral hygiene is important with any type of appliance to avoid tooth decay and gum disease.

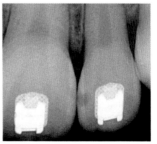

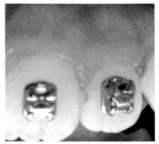

33

Smile Makeover

Here are a few ideas on how to improve a smile. Using 2 or 3 of these options together can make a significant difference.

Cleaning - The first step in having a healthy mouth is having a clean mouth.

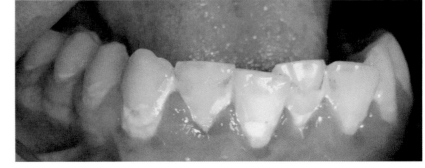

Bleaching - While it doesn't work on calculus or plaque, bleaching works on surface stains like food and coffee. It doesn't work on internal stains like cavities, amalgam or tetracycline. Bleaching doesn't affect any composite fillings, crowns or veneers. Bleach before having any cosmetic work done, so that any new work will match the whiter, bleached teeth.

Clear orthodontic trays can also double as bleaching trays.

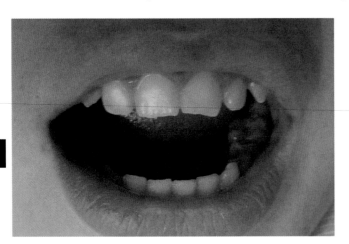
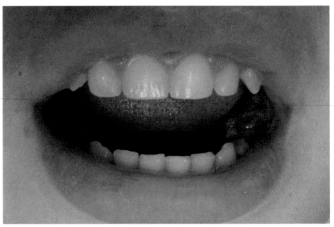

Filing Teeth/Enameloplasty - Sometimes polishing off some rough corners and making all the edges match can make a huge difference.

Periodontal Surgery - Adjusting the gumline can improve a smile.

Braces or Other Orthodontic Appliances - Straightening crooked teeth will not only make them look and feel better, it will make them healthier, be easier to clean and last longer.

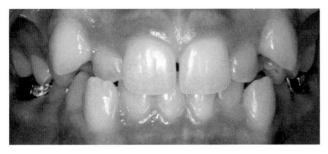 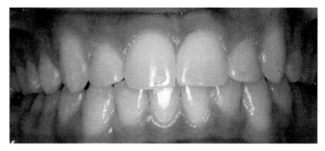

Composite Fillings - Composite restorations can restore cavities, fill spaces, fix broken chips and even make teeth lighter in color.

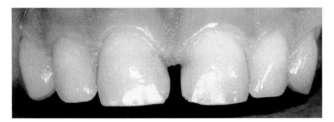 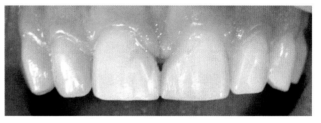

Crowns, Bridges and Veneers - These can cover deeply stained teeth, restore decay and fractures, fix bad spacing and solve other problems.

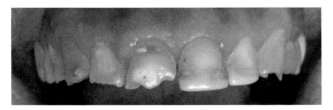 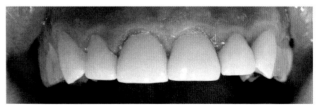

Dentures - There are many temporary and permanent removable options to restore a smile.

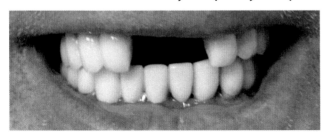 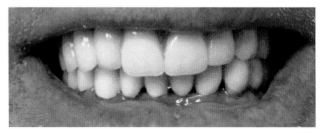

Implants - These can work together with crowns, dentures or braces to help improve a smile.

Sensitive Teeth
Gingival Recession, Exposed Roots

Teeth can become sensitive for any number of reasons such as deep decay, gum disease or trauma. Teeth can also become sensitive when the root surface is exposed. This gingival **recession** normally happens because of over aggressive brushing (scrubbing along the gumline instead of using soft, small movements with a toothbrush).

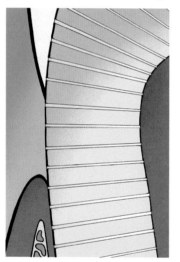

Dentin is filled with little tubes that connect the inside nerve and the outside environment. When the fluid in these tubes move, teeth feel this as sensitivity or pain. The fluid can move because of hot and cold, sweet and sour foods or touching the exposed dentin.

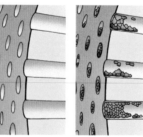

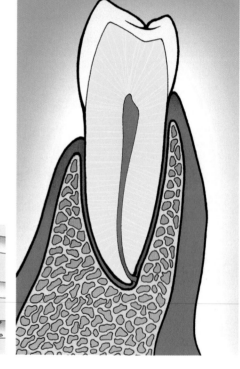

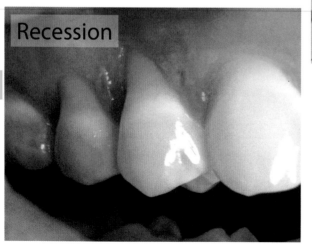

Recession

One way to treat this is to block these tubes so that less fluid can move in and out. Some toothpaste has ingredients that blocks these tubes and makes the nerves less sensitive. The key is to let it sit on teeth, so after brushing do not rinse right away. Do not swallow any toothpaste, spit out the excess and wait a few minutes to rinse.

Clenching
Grinding, Bruxing, Attrition, Abfraction

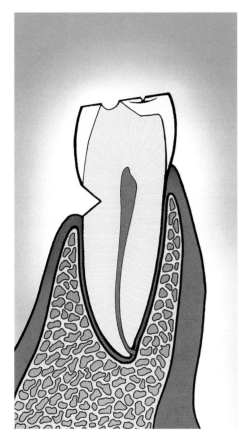

Clenching and grinding causes several things to happen.
Attrition - The teeth wear each other flat on the biting surface. Notice how the softer dentin is worn away faster than the stronger enamel.

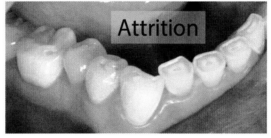

Attrition

Abfraction - As teeth build up tension, they compress and stretch each other as the jaw bone resists this pressure. The result is that the weaker areas along the gumline slowly break apart and wear away, especially those areas not protected by enamel and bone.

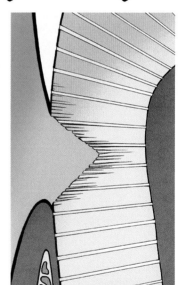

Both of these processes can make teeth more sensitive.

Clenching and grinding (bruxing or bruxism) can happen during the day as a result of stress and can also happen at night. If these habits continue, it is important to wear a **nightguard** to protect the teeth and jaw.

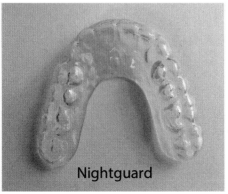

Nightguard

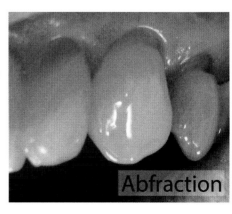

Abfraction

Oral Abnormalities

Examples of some common abnormalities:

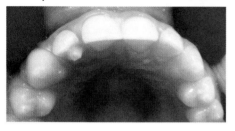

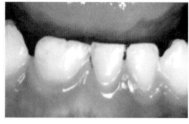

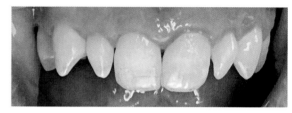

Talon Cusps - An extra cusp that grows on an anterior tooth.

Fused Teeth - Teeth that grow together.

Peg Laterals - The lateral incisors are smaller or misshapen.

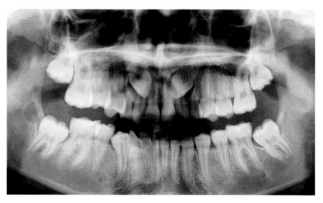

Tetracycline Stain - Taking the antibiotic tetracycline when teeth are forming (up to age 8) can permanently stain them.

Fluorosis - If one ingests excessive fluoride when the teeth are forming, they can grow in with permanent white spots or stain.

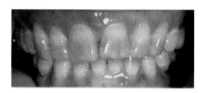

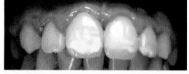

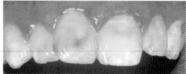

Impacted Teeth - Sometimes teeth don't come in the right way or don't come in at all. This can be corrected with surgery and orthodontics.

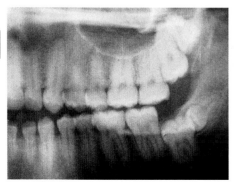

Extra/Missing Teeth - While most people have 20 primary teeth and 32 permanent teeth, some are missing teeth and some have extra. The teeth most often affected are the wisdom teeth.

This person had 8 wisdom teeth.

This person is missing a permanent bicuspid.

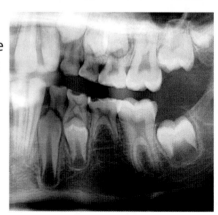

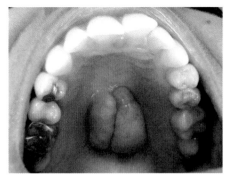
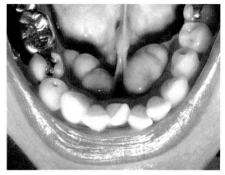
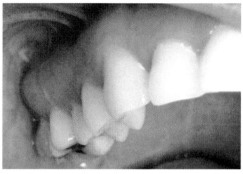

Tori - Extra bone on the inside of the jaw. Tori can be so small that they aren't noticeable, other times they can grow very large.

Bony Extosies - Extra bone on the outside of the jaw.

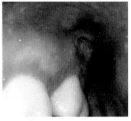
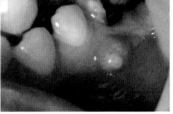
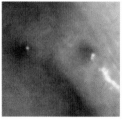
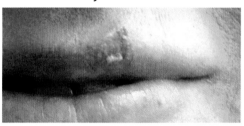

Canker Sore/ Aphthous Ulcer - Usually caused by stress, will normally heal in 2 weeks.

Abscess - These infections can be caused by deep decay, trauma or severe gum disease.

Varix - This is a vein that is close enough to show through the skin.

Cold Sore/Fever Blister/ Herpes Labialis - These are caused by a virus and usually heal in 2-3 weeks.

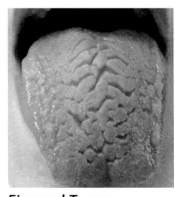
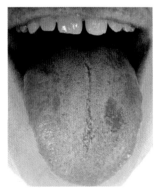
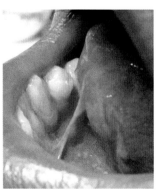
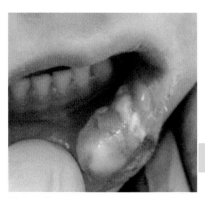

Fissured Tongue - The tongue is covered with deep grooves and fissures.

Geographic Tongue - The tongue has distinctive spots that change over time.

Tongue Tied - The lingual frenulum is unusually short. This can make it difficult to speak.

Post Opperative Trauma - After dental treatment, be sure not to bite or chew any numb areas. This usually doesn't cause any permanent damage.

Dental Trauma
Tooth Emergencies

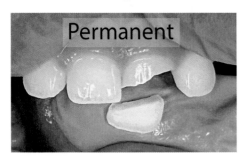

Permanent

After an accident, find out if the teeth involved are primary or permanent.

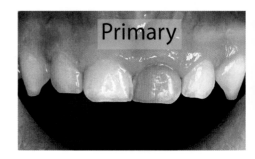

Primary

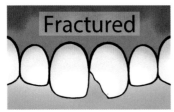

Fractured

Fractured - Look for the tooth fragment, make sure it was not aspirated or swallowed. If it is a large piece, sometimes the dentist can use it. Keep it moist. Visit a dentist within a few days.

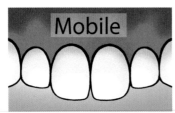

Mobile

Mobile - The tooth is loose, but still in the same position. Don't chew on it and visit a dentist within a few days.

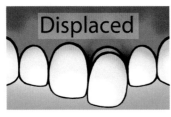

Displaced

Displaced - The tooth is loose, but in a different position. Don't chew on it and visit a dentist immediately.
Do NOT push a primary tooth back in.

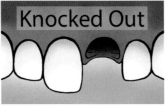

Knocked Out

Knocked out - Look for the tooth. If it is a permanent tooth, pick it up by the crown (the shiny part). Do not touch the root. If it dirty, rinse the tooth in cold running water for 10 seconds. Do NOT scrub the root. Put it back in the socket. If it can't be put back in the socket, place the tooth in the cheek or in a cup with saliva, saline or milk. Do not let the tooth dry out. Do not store it in water. Either will kill the cells on the root. See a dentist immediately. If it is a primary tooth, save it for the tooth fairy.

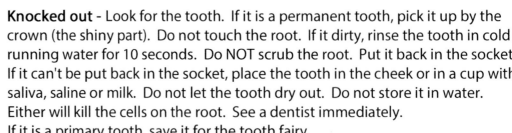

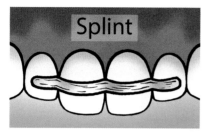

Splint - The dentist may splint a loose tooth to the other teeth using wire or a fiber-reinforced band.

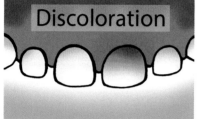

Discoloration - Sometimes when a tooth is injured, it bleeds inside the tooth, turning it dark.

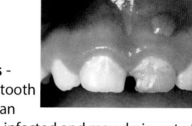

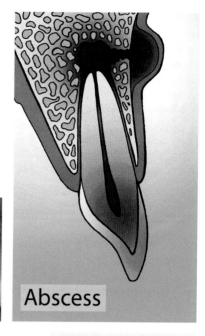

Abscess - When a tooth dies, it can become infected and may drain out of the root. This infection needs immediate treatment.

What do I do After Trauma?

Cracked - When a tooth is cracked, it may just need a filling or smooth out a rough edge. Sometimes the tooth needs a crown, root canal or extraction.

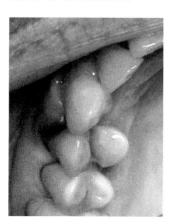

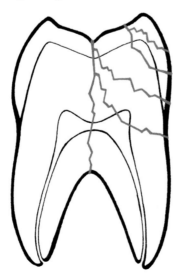

Eat a soft diet for 2 weeks. Do not chew on an injured tooth.

Brush the teeth and tongue with a soft toothbrush, very gently and thoroughly. If there is a splint, it will be difficult to keep clean, but a clean mouth heals faster.

Rinse with salt water or an antibiotic mouthwash after meals and before bed.

Ice and anti-inflammatory medication can help with swelling and pain.

Watch for signs like tooth discoloration or an abscess.

Glossary

Abscess - when an infection is walled off by the body, can drain as pressure builds up

Abutment - the piece that connects the implant to the crown

Amalgam - "silver filling" used for tooth restorations

Anesthesia - a drug that induces a temporary loss of feeling in the body, general or local

Aspirate - to breath something into the lungs

Bicuspids/Premolars - teeth that usually have 2 cusps, the teeth right before the molars

Bond - to adhere something to a tooth micromechanically using composite resin

Bruxism - clenching or grinding teeth

CAD/CAM - Computer-Aided Design/Computer-Aided Manufacturing

Calculus/Tartar - calcified plaque, buildup of bacteria, biofilm and calcium

Canines/Cuspids - teeth next to the incisors, used for tearing food

Carbohydrates, Complex - found in natural sources of whole grains, vegetables, fruits and beans

Carbohydrates, Simple - found in highly processed sources of sugar, white bread, pastries, chips and sodas

Cavity - a hole formed in a tooth by decay

Cement - to adhere something to a tooth using an chemical adhesive, usually an acid/base reaction

Cementum - thin coating on a tooth's root that makes the attachment to bone stronger

Chlorhexidine - an antibiotic used in mouthwash

Composite - "white filling" used for restoration or adhesive, usually cured with a blue light

Dental Appliance - used to aid, replace or protect teeth (braces, bridge, denture, implant, night guard, retainer)

Dental Prosthetic - used to replace teeth, can be fixed or removable (bridge, denture, implant)

Dental Restoration - used to restore a tooth after decay has been removed, direct or indirect (crown, filling, onlay)

Dentin - hard, mineralized material that makes up most of the tooth and root, more flexible than enamel

Enamel - hardest substance made by the body, covers and makes up the crown of the tooth

Enameloplasty - filing, polishing or shaving off some the enamel of a tooth

Fluoride - makes teeth stronger against the acid that bacteria produce

Gingiva - the gums that cover the jawbones and protect the teeth

Implant - the titanium screw that is placed in the jaw, can attach to a crown or denture

Incisor - the teeth in the front of the mouth, used for cutting food and speaking

Lingual Frenulum - the tissue that connects the underside of the tongue to the floor of the mouth

Mandible - the lower jaw

Maxilla - the upper jaw

Metabolize - the process of digesting and absorbing nutrients to sustain life and grow

Molar - large teeth in the back of the mouth, used for grinding food

Periodontal Ligament (PDL) - connects the cementum to the jaw bone

Periodontal Pocket - the pocket at the junction where gingiva wraps around a tooth

Plaque - a sticky buildup of food, bacteria and their waste products, biofilm

Potassium Nitrate - an anti-hypersensitivity ingredient added to toothpaste

Prepare - to remove decay and shape a tooth to receive a filling, crown or root canal

Proxy Brush - a small brush that is useful in cleaning

Pulp - the very inside of the tooth, made up of nerves and blood vessels

Temporomandibular Disorder (TMD) - pain and dysfunction with the TMJ and the associated muscles

Temporomandibular Joint (TMJ) - the joint that connects the mandible to the temporal bone at the base of the skull

Tetracycline - an antibiotic that can cause deep stain in teeth

Tori - extra bone that grows on the inside of the jaw

Xylitol - a sugar that stops the growth of cavity forming bacteria

Dental Specialists

These dentists focus their practice on a specific aspect of dentistry. This normally involves specialized training, extra years of schooling and an additional licensing board. In some cases, these dentists have medical degrees as well. The suffix "dontist" means "tooth doctor," the prefix "oral" means "mouth."

Dentist of Public Health - A dentist who specializes in promoting dental health to the public.

Endodontist - A dentist who specializes in root canals. endo = inside

Exodontist - A dentist who specializes in tooth extractions. exo = outside

Oral Pathologist - A dentist who specializes in diagnosing and treating oral lesions and disease. patho = disease

Oral Radiologist - A dentist who specializes in diagnosing images of the head and neck. radio = x-rays

Oral Surgeon - A dentist who specializes in extractions, impants and jaw surgery.

Orthodontist - A dentist who specializes in braces and moving teeth. ortho = bone

Pedodontist - A dentist who specializes in children's dentistry, a pediatric dentist. pedo = children

Periodontist - A dentist who specializes in gum surgery. perio = around

Prosthodontist - A dentist who specializes in dentures, implants and full mouth reconstruction. prostho = artificial

Tooth Surfaces

The same as how north and south are directions for the earth and right and left are directions for a person, teeth have names for their directions too.

Like a cube has 6 sides, we assign teeth 6 sides and abbreviate them with a letter so that we can communicate about them easier.

Mesial- The side of the tooth that is normally closer to the front of the mouth, adjacent to the next tooth.

Distal- The side of the tooth that is normally closer to the back of the mouth, adjacent to the next tooth.

Buccal (**Facial** or **Labial** on anterior teeth)- The side of the tooth that is normally closer to the cheek, face or lips.

Lingual- (sometimes **Palatal** on maxillary teeth) the side of the tooth that is normally closer to the tongue or palate.

Occlusal (**Incisal** on anterior teeth)- the biting surface of a tooth

Apical- the end of the root, or apex of the root.

Cervical-The middle of the tooth, the thin border that separates the crown from the root.

Interproximal- Between the adjacent surfaces of teeth.

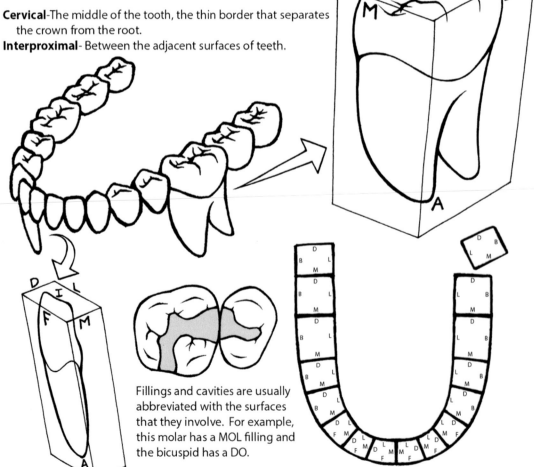

Fillings and cavities are usually abbreviated with the surfaces that they involve. For example, this molar has a MOL filling and the bicuspid has a DO.

Universal Numbering System

The tooth numbering system used most in the United States. The permanent teeth are named with numbers, starting at the patient's upper right. The primary teeth are named with letters.

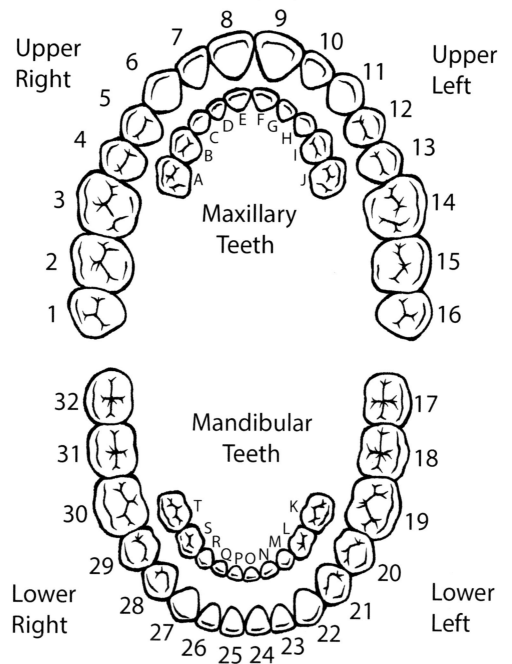

Upper Right

Upper Left

Maxillary Teeth

Mandibular Teeth

Lower Right

Lower Left

Palmer Notation

The tooth numbering system used mostly by orthodontists in the US and dental practitioners in the United Kingdom. The permanent teeth are named with numbers and the primary teeth with letters, both starting at the midline going posteriorly. The teeth are also labeled with an "L" to show the quadrant they are in.

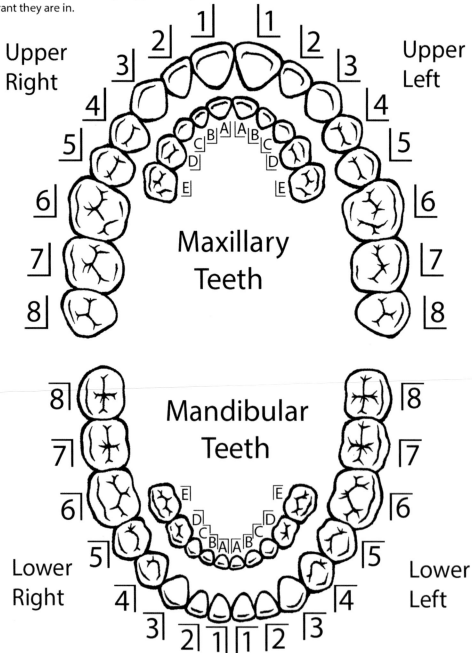

Upper Right

Upper Left

Maxillary Teeth

Mandibular Teeth

Lower Right

Lower Left

FDI Numbering System

The FDI numbering system is the most common tooth numbering system in the world. The teeth are named with two numbers, the first shows which quadrant they are in, the second is the tooth number starting at the midline and going posteriorly. FDI stands for Fédération Dentaire Internationale or the World Dental Federation.

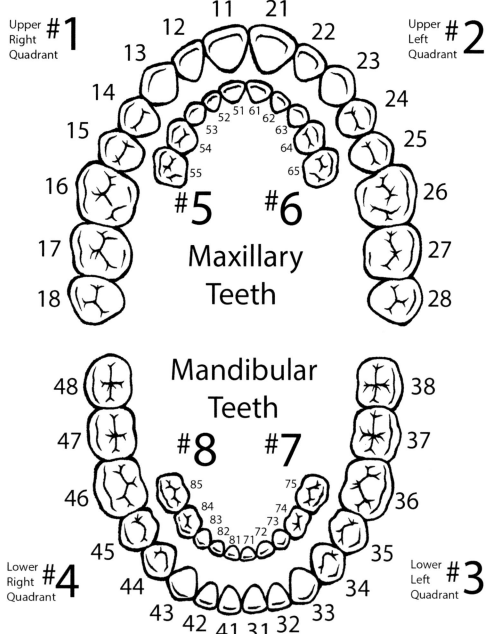

Upper Right Quadrant #1

Upper Left Quadrant #2

Lower Right Quadrant #4

Lower Left Quadrant #3

Maxillary Teeth

#5 #6

Mandibular Teeth

#8 #7

About the Author

Ben Magleby grew up in Portland, Oregon and has always loved drawing. After completing a degree in visual arts at Brigham Young University, he attended University of the Pacific School of Dentistry. Following graduation, Dr. Ben begin his career as an dental officer in the Navy and now practices as a general dentist in California.

Throughout his career, Dr. Ben has enjoyed illustrating a variety of educational materials, including his children's book, *Sugarbug Doug*.

Dr. Ben and his wife have five children. He loves playing and drawing with his kids, spending time with his family and helping others understand a little more about their teeth.

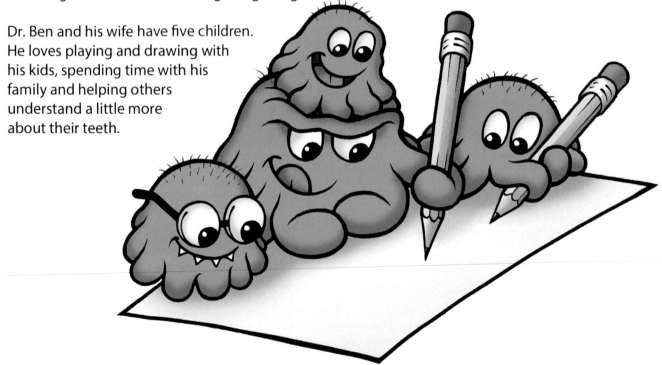

I would like to sincerely thank all of the patients who allowed photographs to be taken for this book. Without your help, this project would never be as good as it could be. I would also like to thank all of the amazing professors at my dental school and all of my outstanding mentors in the Navy. I hope that the examples in these pages capture a small part of the clarity that was taught to me. Last, I want to thank all of my family, friends and colleagues who helped me edit, gather examples and complete this work. Your help is greatly appreciated.

References

Andreasen, Jens Ove Odont Dr. hc. "The Dental Trauma Guide." *http://www.dentaltraumaguide.org/*. 07-01-2014.

Cate, A.R. Ten BDS, BSc, PhD, DSc. *Oral Histology, Development, Structure and Function, 5th Edition.* Mosby. St. Louis, Philadelphia, London, Sydney, Toronto. 1998.

Cohen, Stephen MA, DDS, FICD, FACD and Richard C. Burns, DDS, FICD. *Pathways of the Pulp, 8th edition.* Mosby, A Hardcort Health Sciences Company. St. Louis, London, Philadelphia, Sydney, Toronto. 2002.

Dunlap, Charles, Dr and Dr. Bruce F. Barker. *Oral Lesions, 6th edition.* Colgate Oral Pharmaceuticals. 2002.

Eversole, Lewis R. DDS, MSD, MA, BC. *Clinical Outline of Oral Pathology, Diagnose and Treatment.* Decker Inc, Hamilton. London. 2002.

"Fluoride Toothpaste Use For Young Children." *The Journal of the American Dental Association.* February 2014. pages 190-191.

Garcia, Raul I., Michelle M. Henshaw and Elizabeth A. Krall. "Relationship Between Periodontal Disease and Systemic Health." *Periodontology 2000.* February 2001. Volume 25, Issue 1, pages 21–36.

Jacobsen, Peter L. PhD, DDS. *The Little Dental Drug Booklet.* International Publishing Inc. 2004.

Li, Yiming DDS, MSD, PhD. "An interference with Normal Daily Life." *Dentin Hypersensitivity.* Aegis Communications. September 2013. pages 4-5.

Newman, Michael G. BA, DDS, FACD, Henry H. Takei, DDS, MS, FACD and Fermin A. Carranza, Dr Odont. *Clinical Periodontology, 9th edition.* W.B. Saunders Company. Philadephia, London, New York, St. Louis, Sydney, Toronto. 2002.

Shillingburg, Herbert T. Jr DDS, Sumiya Hobo, DDS, MSD, PhD, Lowell D. Whitsett, DDS, Richard Jacobi, DDS, Susan E. Brackett, DDS, MS. *Fundamentals of Fixed Prosthodontics, 3rd Edition.* Quintessence Publishing Co, Inc. Chicago, Berlin, London, Tokyo, San Paulo, Moscow, Prague, and Warsaw. 1997.

Made in the USA
Coppell, TX
03 November 2023